# To Be or Not To Be:

A Guide to End of Life Medical Decisions

# Thomas Neves

Edited By:
Art Simas

Advice and guidance on publishing by:
Christopher Byron

This book is dedicated to:


My loving and supportive wife, Stacey.

My wonderful children, Haley and Jackson.

All the patients that I have taken care of over the years and their families. Without the experiences we shared together, this book would not have been possible.

The purpose of this book is to educate you about end of life medical decisions. The hope is that, once you have the information, you will be able to make your end of life medical decisions and, most importantly, put them in writing.

A local estate attorney will be able to draft the appropriate legal documents regarding medical treatments. In far too many cases, people must deal with end of life medical decisions at the worst time possible -- when a spouse, parent or another loved one needs that decision made for them. At this point, it may be too late to learn enough about the decisions that you need to make at such a critical time.

Dealing with death is hard enough emotionally and spiritually without having to wade through the various options and corresponding complications of modern medicine. Great technological advances in medicine have been made, but without the proper training, you may not know which medical treatments are necessary or available to you. There are many complicated mechanisms that go into sustaining life, including being kept alive by machines. This book will explain in detail exactly what the medical team will do to keep you or a loved one alive with and without machines. The book will also detail your treatment options in simple, easy to understand terms, and explain the risk vs. reward for each decision. In addition, we'll look at some real life examples of people that made those decisions.

The primary goal is to guide you through a difficult time and encourage you to put your personal decisions in writing, so there is no doubt and no guesswork for anyone. My hope is that you are reading this well in advance of having to make a medical decision, so you can put your wishes in writing and identify a person that can speak on your behalf if you are unable to.

The idea for this book came to me when I was attending to one of my patients. The patient's daughter asked me if I knew of a book that had any information for her, about what her mom was going through. I didn't know of such a resource for caregivers or family members. After many other patients' families asked me the same question, I had to find an answer. I found one book for families about life support and it was written by a medical student in a 380-page textbook that sold for $70. At that point, my mission was clear -- bring complicated life support and end of life issues to the people in language all can understand.

It is intimidating for people to talk with doctors, due in part by the difficult terminology they use. This book will educate you in easy-to-understand language, a minor detail often forgotten by doctors. Whenever complex medical terminology comes into play, I will break it down for the reader. It is very important to know <u>exactly</u> what the doctors are talking about because a misunderstanding may lead to a life or death mistake. I have seen many people with good intentions make poor decisions for themselves or for a loved one on life support. They meant no harm, but they made the wrong decisions because they did not fully understand.

One example of an uninformed decision involved my paternal grandfather. My paternal grandmother became seriously ill and was no longer able to make her own decisions about medical treatment. My grandfather spent nearly all of his time at her bedside, going home only to shower or sleep for a couple of hours at a time. After about two weeks of little to no sleep, my grandfather was asked by the doctor to sign a consent for a surgical procedure. The doctor explained the benefit of the procedure to my grandfather. My grandfather consented to the surgery.

I stopped in for a visit a couple hours later and my grandfather explained to me that he had signed off on the surgical procedure. He told me what he thought the procedure was, but had misunderstood the doctor. In fact, it was nearly the opposite of what the doctor had explained to him. It's not that my grandfather is uneducated; and it's not that the doctor didn't take the time to explain himself. It was the fact that he hadn't been sleeping well, was stressed out, extremely emotional, and he didn't truly understand the terminology the doctor used. Had my grandmother put her wishes in writing, my grandfather would have had a guide to help him make the decisions my grandmother wanted. Eventually, my grandmother had the right procedure done and the doctor was correct. But the point is, my grandfather didn't fully understand what the doctor initially told him.

The opposite situation occurred when my maternal grandfather was diagnosed with pancreatic cancer. He was only 58 and could easily make his own decisions. The doctor spelled out the options for my grandfather and he made up his mind not to treat the cancer aggressively; sadly it was too late. He told the doctor to control the pain and that he wanted to die at home with his family around him. His death was much easier for my mother's family because everyone had peace of mind in knowing they were doing what my grandfather wanted.

You may find yourself in a similar situation to my paternal grandfather. You may have difficulty understanding a doctor. It might be the medical terminology or it may be other factors. I have commonly seen two reasons why people don't understand their doctor:

- The doctor was in a rush and explained the procedure too quickly.
- Many doctors today are born in a foreign country and English is not their first language. Therefore, one may find them difficult to understand.

If you do not fully comprehend what the doctor is trying to explain to you, simply ask him or her to repeat what was said. For instance, you could ask, "Could you repeat that for me one more time, as if I am in sixth grade?" The doctor will understand and take the time to explain things more clearly and thoroughly.

I have found that many doctors are bad communicators. In most cases, doctors simply do not have time to sit with patients ahead of time to discuss the possibility of using various measures that may save their lives. This leads to discussions at a patient's bedside with the spouse or next of kin. And, most often, they must make a decision that is not based on the patient's wishes.

Doctors typically have more than a dozen patients to see and treat at a hospital. How much time do you think he or she will spend talking to families? Not much. With patients and families waiting, an office full of sick people to see, and a bunch of x-rays and other tests to interpret, doctors today have very limited time.

Another common phenomenon is that many doctors encourage aggressive, life-saving procedures that are intended to keep a patient alive at all costs. That is what they learned in medical school.

Here is a scenario: Your mom is very ill with pneumonia and you are visiting her in the hospital. Her doctor decides, because of her high fever and the severity of the pneumonia, your mom is not in the proper state of mind to make her own decisions.

The doctor tells you your mother can't make her own decisions and that you will have to decide for her. The doctor will turn to you and ask you, "If your mother should stop breathing or her heart stops beating, do you want us to do everything we can to try to save her?"

Well of course the answer is yes, save my mom.

Or the doctors will simply ask, "If something happens to your mom, do you want us to try to save her?" But, what if your mom never really wanted *everything* that goes into 'saving' her? What does 'saving her' entail?

There are certain physicians that will, and do discuss the options ahead of time with patients and their families. Other doctors will ask for information at the bedside, as in the scenario just presented. In addition, there may be a language barrier between doctor and patient or the patients loved ones. Doctors are well-educated, well-read and very smart people. It is difficult for them to grasp the idea that not everyone fully understands what they are talking about, because discussing complicated medical terminology is second-nature for them.

But of all the reasons, I felt this type of book will be helpful to those who need guidance and answers. No doubt, this is a very complicated and uneasy subject. But I've seen the anguish on too many faces too many times as they make life or death decisions for someone they have loved for years. It is my belief that the more well-informed a person is, the better decisions he or she will make.

I am not a doctor. If you have specific questions relating to you and your health or medical history, you should call your doctor. My perspective is derived from my 16 years of hands-on experience with death and dying -- and saving lives.

I have a Bachelor of Science Degree in Respiratory Therapy from Quinnipiac University in Hamden, Connecticut. I spent two clinical years, predominantly at Yale-New Haven Hospital, and have been the Primary Therapist on a Respiratory Unit in a community hospital for over 16 years. I have taken care of nearly 1,000 people on life support, and helped their families through the process. It is my job not only to educate the patients and their families, but also to help get the patients well enough so they will no longer need life support. What I share with you is what I have learned along the way. I want you to be informed, so that when the time comes, you will be able to make the best possible decision for you and your loved ones.

Real Life, and Death

I have seen siblings fighting for control of their parent's life. I have seen patients on life support get restraining orders against their families. In another case a gentleman kept his mother alive on life support for over three years, even though she was 'brain dead', simply because he kept on cashing her Social Security checks.

During my career, I have initiated life support and also stopped life support. Removing a person from life support is something that Respiratory Therapists must come to terms with. It's part of the job. Many refuse to remove patients from life support because they feel like they are killing the person. I used to be fearful of it, but the situation has become very common for me after all the years. I've come to realize that the medical community and someone else's decision are artificially keeping the person alive; removing the life support allows nature to take its course. That is not to say that letting nature take its course always means that the person immediately dies. I have seen people die within minutes of the removal of life support, and I have seen people die days or weeks later. I have also removed life support to allow one gentleman to die when he was given no chance to survive. Not only did he live through his rehabilitation, he is still alive and living in his home as I write this book.

On the other hand, being on life support does not mean a person cannot die. That is a common misconception among many people I have met. People can and do die on life support. Because I have seen all of this, I can tell you without an ounce of doubt that the best thing you could ever do for yourself and your family is to be prepared ahead of time. Be as specific as possible about what medical procedures you want and clearly nominate one person to act on your behalf should you become unable to speak or make decisions for yourself.

It is also essential for me to stress that I am not here to try to tell you what decisions you should make. The decision to go on life support is deep, emotionally and spiritually. It is a decision that should be well thought out ahead of time. The life-saving medical procedures covered in this book are the most common procedures we use to save lives. You will be able to use this book as a guide for medical decisions that are right for you. Some examples follow.

A 90 year-old, we will call her Gladys, has been in a nursing home for two years. For the duration of that time, Gladys has had worsening dementia (a condition in which mental ability deteriorates) and now, she doesn't even know her name. Gladys only gets an occasional visitor while in the nursing home and mostly sits in her chair by herself. One day, her heart stops beating and she stops breathing. A staff member happens to be in the room and quickly responds. The nursing staff is able to save 90 year-old Gladys and eventually stabilize her. She is transferred to the local hospital in an ambulance. But upon arrival to the emergency department, her heart is beating, but she is still not breathing. The medical staff immediately places her on a life support ventilator that will breathe for her.

Gladys' next of kin must decide if they should keep her alive with the machine or if they should remove her from life support. In all likelihood, without the machine to breathe for her, Gladys will die. Since Gladys has had dementia for the last two years, her family never got around to asking her if she would want to be kept alive by machines. Her next of kin, two nieces, have differing opinions about life support. One thinks Gladys should be kept alive, the other thinks the machines are just prolonging the inevitable. Until the nieces can come to a mutual decision, Gladys will be kept alive.

Another example of the use of life support is a 30-year-old woman, Joan. Joan has attempted suicide and is found by a family member who calls 911. The paramedics arrive and Joan is revived. Upon arrival at the emergency room, her heart is beating but she is not breathing and she is placed on life support. Further tests reveal there is little brain activity left and she will be a 'vegetable' for the rest of her life.

Joan is now 35. She still has little brain activity and remains on life support today. The decision to initiate life support was made for this family because it was an emergency situation. The family must decide if they will ever want to remove the life support and let nature take its course. The complication in this case is that Joan has two children who were 3 and 4 years old when she attempted suicide. While most of her family agrees that they do not want to keep Joan on life support, they go against their own opinions and keep Joan alive because of her children. The children still go visit mommy in Joan's long-term facility once a week. The rest of the family just doesn't have the heart to let Joan die.

A 20 year-old male, Bill, is having a severe asthma attack and his girlfriend drives him to the hospital. Upon arrival, he is wheezing uncontrollably. His airways slowly squeeze tighter and tighter. Finally, he can hardly breathe. The 20-year-old makes the decision to be sedated and placed on a breathing machine until the asthma attack can be resolved. Without the use of life support Bill will continue to struggle to breathe and may lose his life. Bill's decision is fairly easy for him to make. He grew up with asthma and has learned quite a bit about his disease over the years. Nearly all the time, an asthma attack is reversible with time and the right medications. Bill and the emergency physician know that Bill will probably only require life support for a day or two. After the medicines kick in and the factor that triggered his asthma attack is removed, Bill will be able to breathe on his own once again and life support is removed.

A 55 year-old male, John has a routine knee surgery and spends a couple of days in the hospital for observation. While in the hospital, John develops pneumonia and has increasing difficulty breathing since the operation. Pneumonia is a common side effect of any surgery in which anesthesia is used. That is because anesthesia suppresses your breathing. The suppressed breathing, in conjunction with the fact that John had knee surgery and could not get out of bed, greatly increased his chances of getting pneumonia.

John and his wife are approached by John's doctor when his breathing worsens. The doctor asks John if he wants the staff to try to save him should he stop breathing or his heart stop beating. John and his wife talk about it and come to a decision the day before his breathing deteriorates. He is placed on a breathing machine to ease his difficulty breathing until the pneumonia can be properly treated with antibiotics. When his pneumonia clears up, John can breathe on his own and will no longer needed life support.

In each of the preceding cases, life support and decisions about medical treatments were involved. The message is that there is no clear-cut, correct answer. What you think is appropriate for you is the correct answer. That is why it is so important for you to make your decisions ahead of time and put them in writing. It is your life. It should be your death, too.

It's on Paper, Now What?

   After you make up your mind about which medical treatments you want, what do you do next? This is where the legal aspect comes in. Once you've made your medical decisions, you'll want to have them in writing in some form of legal documentation. The legal document in your state may be referred to as a Health Care Proxy, a Living Will, an Advanced Directive, or a Health Care Power of Attorney. For the purposes of this book, I will refer to the appropriate health care documentation as a Living Will. Your Living Will should clearly state which medical treatments you do and do not want performed. In your Living Will, you may also nominate a person to speak on your behalf and uphold your decisions for you should you become unable. Most people nominate a spouse and that is a logical choice. However, it is also a good idea to nominate a second person to make medical decisions for you should you and your spouse become unable. For instance, if you are in a car crash, your spouse may be in the car with you. Having that second person gives you added peace of mind. Because the laws on medical decisions vary from state to state, consult your local attorney to see which type of documentation is appropriate in your state. Typically, an estate attorney will know the laws in your state and draw up proper medical documentation. However, if you already have a Will,

the attorney that drafted it can probably do your
Living Will.

The life-saving procedures you will learn
about can be separated into four major categories:
breathing, cardiac, the kidneys and food. I'll explain
the medical options for each. At the end of every
category, there will be a quick review you can use
as a checklist of the treatments you think you
might want. I'll finish the medical portion of the
book with some quality of life issues that many
people never consider when making end of life
decisions. Did you know you are more likely to get
an infection in the hospital than you are in public?
Have you ever thought about what it might feel like
to lie in bed for days on end? Ever wonder what it
would be like if you couldn't talk, or couldn't eat?
Those are just some of the things to take into
consideration with quality of life and I'll give you
specific examples of each.

Breathing

The area in your lungs where air moves into your blood is equal to an area the size of a tennis court.

Mrs. Betty Shaw was not your typical 78-year-old woman. Like most, she was worried about her looks, but unlike most, she looked more like 58 than 78. Mrs. Shaw took pride in her looks, keeping up with fashions and never appearing in public without her makeup being just right. Though a widow, she was a social woman with a passion for bridge. She was not only a member of the local bridge club, she was its founder. Every Saturday afternoon like clockwork, you would find Mrs. Shaw at the local Senior Center in the middle of everyone, pairing people up for the bridge matches. Additionally, to help keep her mind sharp, she was involved in a book club.

Mrs. Shaw was very popular among the older gentlemen, but never felt comfortable 'dating' again after her husband passed away. She was much more interested in teaching her 6-year-old granddaughter how to be a lady. Mrs. Shaw was a devout Catholic and never missed church services on Sunday. Of course, it probably goes without saying she was also very good at crochet. However, throughout her life Mrs. Shaw had made one major mistake. She never stopped smoking.

Breathing is the most critical body function in sustaining life. In order to understand the goal of life-saving procedures involving breathing, we need to get a clear understanding of what exactly happens when we breathe.

When we inhale, or take a breath in, we fill our lungs with air. It just so happens that about 21% of that air is oxygen. The breath reaches the millions of tiny air sacks at the end of the airways in our lungs. These air sacks are in close contact with the blood vessels in the lungs. When the air is breathed in, the oxygen automatically "jumps" from the air sacks into the blood vessels. The blood carries the oxygen from the lungs to every other part of our bodies. The cells in our bodies use the oxygen in order to turn food particles into energy. It's a very complicated process that results in energy, but also a waste product called carbon dioxide. Like oxygen, carbon dioxide is a gas found in the air all around us. However, it makes up less than 1% of the air. The blood then carries the carbon dioxide back to the lungs where it "jumps" into the air sacks. When we breathe out, or exhale, we breathe out the carbon dioxide. The entire process can be summarized quite simply as: we breathe in oxygen and breathe out carbon dioxide. The problem is that carbon dioxide, much like the more popular carbon monoxide, is a poison.

So, if we have a problem breathing, the carbon dioxide slowly builds up in the blood and can eventually kill us. If we are going to save someone's life, then we must not only make sure they get enough oxygen, but also make sure the breathing is effective enough to remove the poisonous carbon dioxide.

As I mentioned, Mrs. Shaw smoked for the majority of her life. She began smoking as a teenager, and while in her late 60s it started to take a toll on her body. She developed emphysema and chronic bronchitis. These chronic lung diseases together are known as COPD, chronic obstructive pulmonary disease. Emphysema is the destruction of lung tissue, specifically the air sacs. These tiny alveoli get damaged and group together, trapping air in the lungs. This air can never be breathed out. Bronchitis is the swelling of airways and the phlegm that is produced due to the swelling. Eventually these disease states worsen and the person has a very difficult time breathing.

The most basic means to help someone breathe is by performing mouth-to-mouth resuscitation. In the hospital setting, we don't use our mouths to breathe for the patients that stop breathing. Instead we use what is referred to as an AMBU bag.  The AMBU "bag" is actually made up of three major parts. There is a mask that covers the nose and mouth of the patient, the bladder, which holds the 'breath' which will be given through the mask and finally the reservoir, which holds the reserve oxygen which will fill the empty bladder. The breath is given by squeezing the bladder with the hand, forcing the air out of the bladder, through the mask, into the nose or mouth and into the lungs.

AMBU is not necessarily one of the choices given when it comes to making a Living Will, nor is it an option by itself in the hospital. It is worth mentioning here, because it may very well be a procedure that you would want performed on you should you stop breathing. However, you may not want to proceed to the next step in the breathing portion of saving your life.

The problem with the AMBU bag is that it doesn't ensure the breath gets into your lungs. There are two reasons for this. First, the mask portion may not quite fit your nose and mouth properly. For adults, the mask is one-size-fits-all and is only as good as the person holding it over your nose and mouth. Second, and more importantly, our anatomy makes the AMBU bag inefficient. In our throat, there are two pathways. One, (trachea) leads to the lungs and one (esophagus) leads to the stomach. Therefore, when the mask is held over the nose and mouth and the bag is squeezed, we know the air goes into the nose and mouth. The problem is that we don't know where it goes from there. Chances are most of the air goes into the lungs, but some of it goes into the stomach. It's impossible to say how much of the air actually makes it to the lungs -- and that is not a chance we can take when trying to save your life. The only way to ensure the breath goes into the lungs is to insert a tube into the lungs.

This is where your first decision should be made, so pay close attention; you'll want to know if you would want intubation. The process by which a tube is place through your nose or mouth, down your throat, through your vocal chords and into your lungs is called intubation. The intubation tube is also called an endotracheal, or E.T. Tube. Intubation is the second step in the breathing category of trying to save your life. Typically with this procedure there is no turning back. Once the tube is in place, if you survive the reason why you stopped breathing in the first place, you'll be placed on a breathing machine. In the meantime, while the medical team is still saving your life, the AMBU bag gets connected to the tube in your lungs. We will continue to breathe for you using the AMBU, only through the tube instead of using the mask system.

Intubation is what we would refer to as an invasive procedure. Any time that you have something placed into your body it is considered to be an invasive procedure. For example, an intravenous or IV catheter and a urinary catheter are considered invasive procedures. These invasive procedures can make you susceptible to infections. This is because bacteria that normally wouldn't be able to get through your skin can more easily penetrate through the IV. When we breathe, our bodies heat, humidify and filter the air before it gets to the lungs. Once the intubation tube is placed, it bypasses the body's filtering system and you become more vulnerable to infection. There is always a risk vs. reward for any medical procedure. The risk for the AMBU was getting extra gas in the stomach, which is no big deal, but the AMBU mask is less effective breathing for you than an AMBU with the intubation tube. The reward for using an intubation tube is a secure pathway for the breath to reach your lungs. But the primary risk is infection.

Another risk of having an intubation tube is based on the skill level of the medical professional who places the tube. I've seen intubation tubes placed with ease and I've seen tubes placed with great difficulty. The intubation tube is placed between the vocal chords, so there is the risk of damage to them, and therefore the chance that it affects your voice for the rest of your life should you survive. You should also be aware that intubation generally goes hand-in-hand with a breathing machine.

The breathing machine, sometimes called a ventilator or respirator is considered life support. So when you hear of someone that is on life support, that means a machine is breathing for them. When you stop breathing and the medical team tries to revive you, they will progress from the AMBU, to the intubation tube and, if they are able to save your life, the ventilator will be attached to the intubation tube, for life support.

As I touched on earlier, the common misconception about life support is that it supports all life and you cannot die if you are on a ventilator. A life support system is merely a machine that breathes for you. If your heart stops, the ventilator will continue to breathe for you. If your brain stops functioning, the ventilator will continue to breathe for you. In both cases you may be considered medically 'dead' even though you are on the life support machine. That is one of the biggest misunderstandings that I have come across. Many families believe their loved one on life support will not die simply because they are on life support.

The ventilator is a machine that breathes for you 24 hours a day, 7 days a week, 365 days a year. There are many different types of ventilators made by many different companies, but they all essentially do the same job. Some older ventilators are controlled by valves, springs and air pressure, while most of today's ventilators are controlled by microprocessors and microchips. They have fancy displays and make all kinds of fancy sounds. Ventilators, or Vents for short, are extremely accurate and sensitive. This is important because it is crucial that the vent be precise in delivery and in measurement of breaths.

At this point, I want to take a moment to address those who currently have a loved one on life support. Because a vent is highly sensitive, you may hear it alarm from time to time. This is not something to be overly concerned about. Some minor things may set off the alarms, such as sneezing or coughing. But there are some major issues that will trigger the vent alarms as well. If you notice that the machine has become disconnected from the patient, this IS something to worry about. This renders the vent useless and has technically removed the person from life support. It is essential in most cases that the vent immediately be reattached by the nearest HEALTH CARE PROFESSIONAL. It is most important that you NEVER attempt to reattach the vent yourself and NEVER, under any circumstances should you touch any of the buttons, dials or switches.

Because the machines are so sensitive, your loved one is completely dependant upon them and it is imperative that you not change any of the settings, even by accident. It is life support and you may do serious harm to your loved one.

Once the doctor and medical staff have been able to save you and you are in stable condition, the main goal is to get you healthy enough to successfully be taken off the life support. That's right, as soon as we get you on the ventilator, the staff is working to remove it. Something major has obviously happened to you if you need a ventilator. There are numerous causes, but there is no need to elaborate in this book. The point is, the medical team will get to work on whatever caused you to need a ventilator as soon as possible. This is because, generally speaking, the longer you are on life support, the harder it is to get off life support.

Breathing on Your Own

Breathing is something we don't normally think about while we are healthy. The muscles we use to breathe are similar to other muscles in the fact that, when they are not used, they get small and weak. Have you ever broken your arm or leg or known someone who has? Did you see what happened to your muscles when they weren't being used? That's right, they got small and weak. The same thing happens to people on life support. While the machine is breathing for them, they don't use their breathing muscles. The muscles become weakened or atrophied and then it becomes more and more difficult to breathe without the help of the machine. I'll give you a personal example.

When I was new to the field, a medical representative was selling us a new product. It was a breathing machine that did not require an intubation tube. Rather, it used a mask over the nose and mouth similar to how AMBU works. The rep was preparing to give his talk on how the machine is beneficial and asked for a volunteer to try it. Without hesitation I raised my hand. I wanted to know what my patients would go through on such a machine. Of course, no one else volunteered so I was picked. After properly fitting the mask over my nose and mouth, the rep turned the machine on. It was a strange feeling to have air blown into my lungs. Actually, it is backwards from the way that nature intended. When we breathe, our diaphragm moves down creating a negative pressure (vacuum) in our lungs so air gets sucked in. The diaphragm automatically moves back into its original position and we breathe the air out. While on a breathing machine, no negative pressure, or vacuum is created. Rather, the air is just forced into the lungs, which causes positive pressure. Anyway, it took a good 5 to 10 minutes for me to get used to the machine, but I was able to finally get comfortable. For the rest of the presentation I felt very relaxed and comfortable, to the point where I probably could have taken a nap. The machine just kept giving breaths and I was receptive to them. It was when the presentation was over that I ran into problems. The rep finished up and turned the machine off as I removed the mask.

Now, I have always been active and physically fit. At the time I was about 25 years old, playing hockey three to four times a week, and working out at the gym. I was in what I would consider to be great shape.

However, when I removed that mask I could not catch my breath. When I tried to breathe in, nothing happened. I tried again and got no air. It took all I had to move just a little air into my lungs. This went on for a good minute or two before I felt normal again. The point being, if a physically fit person gasps for air after only 30 minutes on a breathing machine, imagine what it must be like for someone that is sick to begin with and on a breathing machine for a week or more.

Besides the breathing muscles weakening, there are other factors to consider about life with a breathing machine. First, because the intubation tube is between your vocal chords, you cannot talk. Everything that you have to communicate will have to be written down. Second, you cannot eat. There is a big tube in your nose or mouth and swallowing properly is impossible, so the doctors don't even try to feed you. It is more complicated than just feeding you, so I'll save the details for the FOOD section.

You may be awake and alert while on the ventilator or the doctor may choose to sedate you to ensure that you won't pull the intubation tube out. Obviously, it is not natural to have a tube in your lungs and your natural tendency is to want to pull it out. To prevent this, the staff may have to restrain your arms. Again, for your own good you may have your arms tied to the bed just in case you wake up in the middle of the night and try to pull the tube out. Think about your children or grandchildren coming in to visit you. You'll have a tube in your nose, won't be able to speak with them and you may be tied to the bed.

In addition to all that, the staff is going to have to "suction" your intubation tube. By suction, I literally mean, put a smaller catheter through the intubation tube and vacuum out any secretions you may have in your lungs. Because the intubation tube is considered by your body to be a foreign invader, your body attacks it. That means you make more saliva, phlegm and or sputum in and around the tube. These are fluids that can't be allowed to remain in your lungs or they'll cause pneumonia, so the medical team must vacuum them out. I've suctioned people as infrequent as every three hours and as frequent as every half hour depending on the severity. While suction is not painful, it feels just like choking on something you swallowed down the wrong pipe, so I wouldn't say it's comfortable. The good news is that you are alive.

You are alive and there may be hope for recovery. When you start to breathe on your own again and you no longer need the ventilator, the intubation tube can be easily removed. What a relief! You can probably talk again immediately, but you will have quite the sore throat and your voice may not sound normal for some time.

That is the good scenario, but what if you are not getting much better and are having a difficult time breathing on your own?

If you are not successfully breathing on your own and require the ventilator for the foreseeable future you will have yet another decision to make. Thus far you have agreed to intubation and mechanical ventilation, the next decision will come about two weeks after you have been intubated.

The generally accepted amount of time that you can safely have an intubation tube in your vocal chords is about two weeks. After that, it is possible for your vocal chords to become paralyzed because of the tube. Vocal chord paralysis not only means that you may never talk again, but also that you may not be able to live without an artificial airway of some sort. Long before we get to that stage, your doctor will approach you about that third decision, a tracheostomy.

A tracheostomy is a surgical procedure in which the doctor makes a hole in the center of your neck below the vocal chords, directly into your windpipe, which in medical terms is a trachea. As far as medical terminology is concerned, any time the word ends in "-ostomy" it means a hole. Tracheostomy is a hole in the trachea. Colostomy is a hole in the colon. Whenever the term ends in "-ectomy" it means removing something. A tonsillectomy is the removal of the tonsils; a splenectomy is the removal of the spleen. Let's get back to your tracheostomy shall we?

A tracheostomy is performed by a surgeon while you are under anesthesia. The hole is cut into your windpipe and a shorter version of the intubation tube is placed in the hole. The new tube is called a tracheostomy tube, or trach (rhymes with lake) for short. Once again you must consider your risk vs. reward for this procedure. Anytime you have a surgery there is risk, but when you have surgery on your neck it is extremely risky. The surgeon must be precise or you may bleed to death on the table. You cannot and should not, however, keep the intubation tube through your vocal chords or risk vocal chord paralysis.

You can avoid this situation totally and I have seen people avoid it. They simply put in their Living Will that, should they be unable to breathe without the help of the ventilator after two weeks, they wish to have the ventilator removed regardless of outcome. They give themselves the two weeks with the life support to get well and if they aren't well, then they want to let nature take its course. There is another school of thought, however.

Some studies have shown that it is easier to breathe through the trach tube than through an intubation tube. Therefore, you may be able to successfully "wean" from the ventilator if you have a tracheostomy. I'll show you why with a simple demonstration:

1. Get yourself an ordinary drinking straw.
2. Now breathe only through that straw. Not so easy is it.
3. Now cut the straw in half and you will breathe through it much easier. That is almost exactly the reason why the trach tube is more effective, a shorter tube is easier to breathe through.

Life with the tracheostomy tube is not all that bad once you get used to it. First and foremost, it can be removed if you no longer need it and the hole will close up remarkably quick. Second, you may be able to talk and you may be able to eat! Many people even go home with a trach tube in place. Trach tubes can be taken out and cleaned or replaced. On the flip side, they can be very messy. It is very common for phlegm (pronounced flem) and blood to leak around the trach tube through the hole until it is fully healed. Therefore, thorough cleaning must constantly be performed to prevent infection. I think that sums up tracheostomy, the most invasive of the procedures to save your life in the breathing category.

That leads me to the least invasive and often involuntary breathing procedure, the BiPAP machine. If you think back to my little story about being on the breathing machine and that I had a hard time breathing afterwards, the BiPAP is the machine that was breathing for me. It is noninvasive because it breathes for you via a mask, rather than a tube down your throat. It is often involuntary because it is not considered life support by law, so even if you specify that you do not want breathing machines, the doctor can use a BiPAP on you anyway. That is why I am putting BiPAP in this book.

Like a ventilator, a BiPAP is a machine that breathes for you 24 hours a day, seven days a week, 365 days a year. The only difference being that a BiPAP does not require a tube or intubation. Rather, a BiPAP mask covers your nose and mouth with straps around your head to hold the mask in place. Ideally a BiPAP is used for people, like Mrs.

Shaw, with chronic lung diseases. Because they cannot breathe sufficiently to remove enough carbon dioxide, they sometimes need assistance. So a person with lung disease usually sleeps with a BiPAP mask on in order to breathe the carbon dioxide back to normal levels. They wake up feeling refreshed, but as they go through their daily activities, the carbon dioxide slowly builds back up. When the person goes to bed, they wear the BiPAP again and start the cycle all over again. In these situations, BiPAP improves quality of life.

Without the assistance of BiPAP, carbon dioxide builds up in the blood because we have not been breathing effectively, we lose consciousness, fall asleep and eventually die. However it is not always used that way. Let's look at a common example of how a doctor might use BiPAP in an end of life situation.

You are 80 years old and have had a great life. You are in the hospital with pneumonia and have decided that you do not want to be intubated nor placed on life support. The pneumonia impairs your ability to breathe well enough to remove carbon dioxide and you lose consciousness. The nurse notices that you are unconscious, still breathing and your heart statistics seem normal. The nurse calls your doctor to report that you are unconscious, and the doctor orders BiPAP for you. The nurse writes the order and a BiPAP machine is brought to your bedside to breathe for you via a mask over your nose and mouth, strapped around your head. The BiPAP is now breathing for you and keeping you alive just as a ventilator would.  Just like life support.

However, there is no legislation in place that recognizes BiPAP as life support, so even though you didn't want to be kept alive artificially, there may be nothing you or your family can do about it at that point.

That is why I have included BiPAP here. You may specify what your wishes are about BiPAP in your Living Will. Maybe the idea of being kept alive without having tubes inserted seems like a good idea to you. Maybe you want to specify that you don't want BiPAP or a ventilator. As I have said and will probably continue to say, whatever you choose is the right thing. I merely would like you to be informed about these things ahead of time, so you can logically decide what type of medical treatment you may want.

Poor Mrs. Shaw, you've forgotten all about her. One day her chronic lung disease flared up and she couldn't breathe. She called 911 and was brought to the emergency department. She always told her daughters that she didn't want to be kept alive by machines. However, when it came down to the situation where she was literally gasping for air, suffocating to death, her doctor intervened. He told Mrs. Shaw that if she let him put her on the ventilator he could get her through this episode and back off the ventilator within a few days. With her life in the balance and the panic that sets in when you cannot breathe, she agreed.

I'd like to include a personal thought here if I may. This scenario proves my point about doctors and how they try to save everyone no matter the situation. However, even though Mrs. Shaw never wanted to be placed on life support she had a hard time refusing it when the reality of her own death set in. It is one thing to read this book to try to decide what you would want for treatment. It is another thing entirely when, sometime in the future, it is you that cannot breathe. Hopefully, you can make the right decision for yourself and your loved ones, but realize that situations may change when you're in the hot seat. I can easily say right now, for instance that I would never want to be on life support. I've seen too much, I know too much. Ask any nurse or respiratory therapist if they'll use life support. I'll bet I know what they'll say. However, it is NOT me on the table, it is NOT me struggling to breathe. I just hope that I am never put in that position because I don't know how I'll react.

We'll end our breathing chapter with Mrs. Shaw's progression through the breathing decisions. As we know, she consented to the breathing tube and the breathing machine because her doctor assured her it would only take a few days to get better. After two weeks on the breathing machine (ventilator), Mrs. Shaw and her daughters decided that they should go forward with the tracheostomy procedure. They were told that it would be easier for Mrs. Shaw to breathe and she would be more likely to wean from the ventilator. Shortly after having the trach tube surgically placed, Mrs. Shaw was transferred to the respiratory unit where I first met her and her daughters. By that time, she already had an infection in her tracheostomy. Of course, when you're in the hospital, you don't usually get a 'regular' bacterial infection, and neither did Mrs. Shaw. She was infected with a bacteria called MRSA, we pronounce it as "Mersa." MRSA is a bacteria that is resistant to most antibiotics, which means we can do very little to stop the infection except to treat its symptoms. Once you've got MRSA, you hardly ever get rid of it. Nevertheless, we moved forward and exercised Mrs. Shaw's breathing muscles everyday, a process called weaning. She was doing quite well actually, spending hours at a time without the breathing machine and then 'resting' with the breathing machine to let her muscles recuperate.

Then, one day Mrs. Shaw changed. She became extremely anxious. She went from spending most of the daytime without the ventilator to just a couple hours a day without it. Then she would only tolerate a few minutes without the ventilator until finally she could not come off the machine at all. Mrs. Shaw's 'couple of days' on the ventilator that her doctor had promised her turned into a little more than two years before she finally passed away.

Your "Breathing" Checklist:

Now that we've covered these medical treatments that assist with breathing, it is time to make your choice. Which of the following will you want and which do you prefer not to have?

>AMBU
    (the bag that simulates mouth to mouth resuscitation)

>BiPAP
    (the machine that breathes for you without a tube)

>Intubation
    (the tube in your mouth and vocal chords)

>Ventilator
    (breathing machine with intubation tube)

>Tracheostomy
    (hole in neck with shorter breathing tube)

Cardiac

Your heart beats about 100,000 times per day and 35 million times per year. Over your lifetime, your heart will beat 2.5 billion times!

Mr. Jones was a 52-year-old man whose father had died of a heart attack at age 58. Mr. Jones was a man's man as they say. He smoked cigars, drank beer, and worked in the construction industry. He was a rough, tough, mountain of a man. His mantra was that people shouldn't try to tell him what to do or how to live his life. He would always ask, "What do they know?" And, "I could drop dead tomorrow, so why should I change my lifestyle?" This reckless attitude was the cause of much grief for his wife.

In this chapter you will learn about the different medical procedures involving your heart. There are many life-saving procedures for the heart -- too many to cover in this book. To make things easier, we'll focus on the ones that are used in an emergency, when your heart stops. We'll stick with those situations because you won't be able to make a decision if your heart stops. On the other hand, some treatments, such as angioplasty or bypass surgery, allow for some time to weigh the options and decide whether or not to have them performed. Still others, such as irregular heartbeats, may be treated with pacemakers and drug therapy. Again, there is time in those situations to do some research, talk to the doctor and then make your best decision.

The cardiac treatments that follow will be explained, assuming you are already in a hospital environment or a similar setting in which there is staff that can perform them. Otherwise, if your heart stops in the mall for instance, you won't be given a choice and the life-saving, cardiac procedures will be performed by paramedics or passers-by. You can probably imagine why then, that I want to teach the procedures as they would happen in the ideal setting. Not only is the staff well-trained, but they will also have the right equipment to get the job done. That is, of course, assuming that you want the cardiac medical treatments performed in the first place.

Once again, I am not a doctor and what I will share with you is based solely on my experience with the life-saving procedures covered in this chapter. If you have a question in regard to your specific medical condition you should contact your physician. In such a case, using this book as a guideline to determine what questions you have for your doctor might be a good idea. My hope is that you will feel more comfortable with life-saving cardiac procedures and the knowledge I share about them to be able to make the best decision for you and your loved ones.

In order to understand the procedures used to revive the heart, we must first get a clear understanding of exactly what happens when the heart beats. As we learned, the blood carries oxygen to our cells and the cells use the oxygen to turn food into energy. The blood gets to the cells because of the heart. When the heart beats, it pumps the blood through arteries (big blood vessels) and capillaries (little blood vessels) where the oxygen can reach the cells. Therefore, the heart is just a pump that was designed to move oxygen. The small, upper chambers of your heart contract (beat), sending blood into the larger, lower chambers. Then the lower chambers beat, pumping the blood out of your heart to your lungs and the body. The next logical question would be to ask what makes the heart beat.

The heart beats because it has its own electrical system. The electrical system is made up of special heart cells that generate an electric impulse. The electric system on the heart fires this electric impulse from a node on the upper chambers of your heart. Because the impulse is fired, the upper chambers contract, squeezing the blood into the lower chambers. From the upper chambers, the impulse travels down a series of special heart cells that conduct the electrical impulse to the lower chambers. When the impulse reaches the lower chambers they contract, pumping the blood out of the heart to your lungs and body. It is easy to see that the electrical system is also critical to sustain life.

Now that you have a very basic understanding of how the heart works, it will be easier to understand the cardiac procedures that are used to save your life. The procedures are chest compressions, defibrillation and cardiac medication. Once again, you only have the opportunity to pick and choose which of these therapies you will want performed on you ahead of time. Unless otherwise specified, all of these medical procedures will be performed to keep you alive.

There are many reasons why your heart would stop beating, once again too many to even begin to cover here. The point is that the heart has stopped. When that happens, the first thing that is performed is called chest compressions. Chest compressions are done to simulate your heartbeat as part of CPR, when your heart is not beating. Typically two hands are used in order to perform effective chest compressions. This is done by putting one hand on top of the other using the heel of the bottom hand to press down on the breastbone, known as the sternum, in the upper center of your chest. By pressing the sternum down by 2 inches, the heart gets compressed. Because the heart gets squished, the blood in the heart has no place to go but into your arteries, thereby simulating the pumping action of the heart. Since your heart naturally beats about 60 to 100 times every minute, the goal is to try to do 80 to 100 compressions per minute. Chest compressions are needed in order to circulate oxygen to your body and brain. As we learned earlier, without oxygen, cells die. Obviously we want to save as many brain cells as possible in this situation. The compressions are performed until the next step in the process can be started, defibrillations.

Getting back to our risk/reward theme, there are risks associated with having chest compressions done. Because the sternum is pressed down to nearly 2 inches, a large amount of pressure is exerted on the ribs. The most common complication associated with chest compression is broken ribs. It is easy to understand when you know what is actually happening during resuscitation, even in a hospital setting. An entire medical team rushes to the bedside and many are filled with adrenaline. One of the team members, typically a strong male but not always, starts with the chest compressions. Adrenaline flowing, doctors watching and a life in the balance make for some enthusiastic compressions. Additionally, the doctors will feel for a pulse to make sure that the compressions are strong enough. Would you want to be the team member that gets told your compressions are not good enough in front of everyone else? Also, just how far down *is* 2 inches anyway? I'll bet my idea of 2 inches is different from your idea of 2 inches. Even with the complication of broken ribs, compressions are a necessity because severe brain damage or even death can occur. The chest compressions are done to simulate the heartbeat until the medical team can get your heart

started again. This is where the defibrillator comes
in.

As you learned, the heart beats because of
the electrical impulse. When your heart has
stopped, a most likely cause would be that this
impulse is either firing improperly or not firing at
all. When your heart is defibrillated, a jolt of
electricity is sent through the chest and heart in
hopes of restarting it. Thus, defibrillating a person
is sometimes called "shocking" them. Sending a
large electrical current through the heart can shock
the electrical system, hopefully causing it to reset
and send the normal electric signals. In most cases,
defibrillation is the best way known to get the heart
started again. Therefore, the sooner the heart gets
shocked, the better chance of survival.

That is why you have seen or may see
defibrillators in public places. The technology has
increased to the point where the AED (automated
external defibrillator) can be attached to the person
and then tell the bystanders what to do. Again, the
sooner we can get the heart started the better, so if
bystanders can shock the heart, there is no need to
wait for an ambulance to show up.

To review how we got here, let's look at how it
would go in the hospital setting.

Your heart stops and the staff rush into your
room and first take care of your breathing. Then a
staff member will begin compressions while another
attaches the defibrillator pads. These days we tend
not to use the paddles you have probably seen on
TV. Rather, we put very sticky pads on the chest
and back, and the shock is delivered through the

pads. The pads also record the rhythm of the heart so the docs and staff can determine what's going on. If there is no rhythm, the person is shocked. The amount of electricity used to defibrillate usually starts around 200 Joules (J) for the first attempt and increases to 300J for the second try and then maxes out at 360J for the remaining attempts.

However it is not uncommon for the defibrillation to begin at 360J. That's a lot of electricity. Some people have compared being shocked to being kicked hard in the chest with a big boot. I had one doctor tell me that 360J is enough power to start a diesel truck engine. It just so happens that most people are unconscious at the time and don't have much of a recollection of the event. The shock is also something that Hollywood sometimes overdoes. You may have seen movies or TV shows in which a patient was shocked and the body bounced into the air. That is pretty rare in my experience, though a smaller, petite person may be moved quite a bit by the shock.

Let's take a look at risk/reward for defibrillation. Once again, the obvious reward is staying alive, though defibrillation doesn't always work. One of the risks would be the pain endured by being shocked with electricity. Another risk is that of being burned. While it is rare, if the paddles or pads are not placed correctly, the electricity will not travel through you. Rather, it will burn you. Some other risks include injury to the heart muscle, abnormal heart rhythms and blood clots.

Again, since the alternative is likely death, you may feel it is worth tolerating these risk factors.

If you do not like the idea of being electrocuted if your heart stops, but you'd like them to try something else, cardiac medications are for you. In a typical case, the medical team will also use heart medications to restart your heart in addition to defibrillation. There are too many heart medications and they are just too complicated for me to go in depth. The general idea behind most of the cardiac drugs is to work with your own nervous system. You probably know about your automatic "fight or flight" response to danger. If not, it goes something like this. You are walking through the woods and come across a bear. Your nervous system kicks some adrenaline up causing a "fight or flight" response. You will either fight for your life or run for your life (it might also make you soil your pants). Anyway, the cardiac medications are designed to stimulate or suppress that same nervous system response, based on your situation. In general, the hope is that your body responds to the meds and will change your heart rate, increase the strength of your heartbeat, open the blood vessels to your heart and brain, and decrease the flow of blood to the arms and legs. As mentioned earlier, these medications are typically used in conjunction with defibrillation. The cardiac medications themselves are not as likely to revive you as defibrillation. This is very important for you to understand.

Cardiac meds by themselves are not as successful as defibrillation. Therefore, choosing to use just cardiac meds and not defibrillation decreases the chance that you will survive.

Also, if you decide against compressions, it makes no sense to agree to cardiac medications. The compressions circulate your blood. The cardiac meds are given into your veins. So, if you get medications and the medical staff does not circulate your blood with compressions, the meds will never reach your heart. Therefore the meds will be useless.

The risk reward for using cardiac medications to help revive your heart will be short. The meds are great to support other life-saving procedures, but may or may not be responsible for saving you. So the reward remains staying alive. The risk list is pretty short, unless the medications are mismanaged by your medical team. An overdose or a mistake in giving one of the drugs could kill you. The medications may also cause thyroid problems, liver problems and even swelling in the lungs.

That pretty much wraps it up for the generally accepted treatments that are used to save you should your heart stop beating. Now let's sum up. Obviously, all three used together gives you the best chance of survival. The sooner you are defibrillated, the better your chance for survival. The compressions and cardiac meds just help until the defibrillation can be performed. Now that the medical team has your heart beating again, you may be given some choices about maintaining your new cardiac lifestyle.

Once you have been stabilized and your heart is beating again, the doctors may need to perform other procedures. One of the most common is a cardiac catheterization. Another is the addition of a pacemaker or internal defibrillator. In severe cases they may also need to do bypass surgery. Since these procedures happen after you are stabilized, you and your loved ones will most likely have time to discuss each with your doctor. Therefore, they do not fit within the scope of this book.

Mr. Jones was admitted to my ward because he had a pretty bad pneumonia. He was having trouble breathing and couldn't go to work, so his wife forced him to go to the emergency room. Mr. Jones was very lucky that he listened to his wife. While on my ward, he was being treated for pneumonia with antibiotics through an Intra Venous (IV) line. It was just coincidence that he was about to have a heart attack. I remember I was sitting in the nurse's station documenting on one of my other respiratory patients when Mrs. Jones came out of his room screaming that something was wrong. Upon rushing in, we noticed Mr. Jones was turning blue and wasn't breathing. I immediately began breathing for him with the AMBU bag, while the nurse called for the emergency team. Once I got some breaths in Mr. Jones, I looked up to notice his poor wife coming back into the room to see what was wrong. At this time the rest of the emergency team showed up and Mrs. Jones was escorted to the waiting room.

As the process goes, we started by checking for a pulse. Mr. Jones' heart was not beating. As I mentioned, he was a BIG guy. Because of this, one of the nurses took over the breathing so I could do the compressions. First, it was easier for me to reach over his chest and second, it was going to take some power to give him compressions. Things like this little swap happen all the time with little or no actual talking. The nurse took one look at him, then at me. I offered up my AMBU bag and we switched places. I have to say that I am typically careful with my compressions because I hate to break ribs, but I was pushing pretty hard on Mr. Jones' chest. One of the doctors, while waiting for a reading of the electrical signal of the heart, was checking for a pulse. A nurse was busy applying the defibrillator pads around my handy work. To my surprise the doctor told me I needed to give stronger compressions. The electric signal from the heart came in and the doctor decided to defibrillate. Again, because of the size of Mr. Jones, the doctor decided to start at the maximum level of 360 Joules. The shock was given and I watched the electrical rhythm waver and start to resemble a normal wave before going flat again. I got right back to work on the compressions while the defibrillator recharged. The nurses, under the instruction of another doctor, were starting to inject the cardiac medications into Mr. Jones' IV line. My compressions were the key to get those meds circulated. Then it was another shock, some more compressions and more cardiac meds without any change to his heart rhythm, it was still flat. I was sweating profusely as I worked the compressions, I remember because I cringed as I watched the sweat drip on top of the defibrillator pad, but to my relief, nothing happened. Mr. Jones was getting close to the end. Then a third shock at 360 Joules and the heart rhythm fluttered, bounced and then normalized. His heart was beating on its own again. He was probably going to make it. That was the last I saw of Mr. or Mrs. Jones, as he was rushed to the cardiac care unit. One of my co-workers told me Mr. Jones walked out of the hospital on his way home just two weeks later. Hopefully, he learned his lesson, but something tells me he hasn't changed much.

Your "Heart" Checklist:

Now that we've covered the medical treatments that assist and revive the heart, it's time to make your choice. Which of the following will you want and which do you prefer not to have?


>Compressions
      (a person pushing down on your chest)

>Defibrillation
      (shocking your heart with electricity)

>Cardiac Meds
      (help change the way the heart pumps)

## Kidneys

Your kidneys can process over 30 gallons of fluid in 24 hours.

Mr. Wayne was a 49-year-old mentally retarded patient. He was admitted to my ward from his long-term care facility with acute respiratory failure. He had been on a ventilator for almost two years and had a tracheostomy tube. I remembered him from when his initial breathing problems began two years earlier. He was a joyful man who loved to joke around. When I'd go in and call him by his real name he would joke, "No, I'm Batman!" It was nice to see Mr. Wayne again, but he was not the same guy he had been. The ventilator was helping Mr. Wayne breathe, but for some reason unknown to the staff at his facility, he was breathing too fast. When we did our work-up on him, his blood work was not normal. Further testing revealed that Mr. Wayne's kidneys were starting to fail.

In this brief chapter we will focus on the kidneys. Again, this is not my specialty and should you have problems with your kidneys you will probably be seen by a kidney doctor. A Nephrologist is a doctor that specializes in the kidneys and will help you determine what treatment is best for you

and how often you will receive treatment. This
chapter will give you a basic overview and should
provide you enough information, based on my
experiences, to decide if the treatments for kidney
failure are treatments you will want.

The kidneys are also essential to sustain life.
In most cases kidney failure, also known as renal
failure, is a long process. There is typically a lot of
time to get educated about treatments for and
prevention of kidney failure. There are some cases,
however, where the kidneys fail quickly and there is
not a lot of time to make decisions. It is for these
times that I have included the kidneys in this book.
It's probably something that people should include
in their Living Will, regardless of long onset or in an
emergency. Once again, before we learn about how
renal failure will be treated, it will help to know a
little bit about what exactly the kidneys do.

The main job of the kidneys is to filter the
blood. As blood passes through the kidneys, it is
filtered and the waste products are extracted. They
also remove fluid from the blood if necessary. This
fluid, along with the waste products removed from
the blood, become urine. Another job of the kidneys
is to help keep the proper chemical balance in the
blood. For instance, the kidneys can add calcium if
blood levels of calcium are low; and they can
remove calcium if the blood levels are too high. The
kidneys also tell the body to make new blood cells,
help control blood pressure, regulate blood pH
(acidity,) and help keep bones strong.

As you can see, the kidneys have a huge
impact on the proper function of your body.  If the

kidneys suddenly fail there will be a number of side effects, most of which are life threatening. There is no cure for kidney failure, so when the kidneys fail, we must replace them or find another way to filter your blood. The only way to filter your blood without the aid of kidneys is a process called dialysis.

Dialysis is the process of artificially filtering your blood. There are two types of dialysis that are generally used, peritoneal (pronounced perry-ton-eel) dialysis and the more invasive hemodialysis. It should be noted here that either dialysis may be used in emergency situations other than renal failure. Dialysis in general, has been used to treat poisoning and drug overdose. Peritoneal dialysis has also been used to treat heat stroke by using dialysis fluid that has been chilled.

Peritoneal dialysis is the least invasive dialysis procedure. This procedure involves filling your abdomen with dialysis fluid. There is a sack in your abdomen called the peritoneal membrane that contains your stomach and intestines. It is this sack that gets filled with the dialysis fluid. In order to have peritoneal dialysis an incision is made, typically on your stomach and a catheter is placed through the incision. If peritoneal dialysis is going to be done regularly, the catheter will be stitched into place and will not be taken out in between treatments. Once the catheter is placed in the abdomen, a dialysis fluid is poured in and the catheter gets closed. Two to three liters of dialysis fluid is the typical amount. You can probably easily picture a two liter bottle of soda, so then you can understand that at least that much dialysis fluid will be used each time. The fluid is left in the abdomen for approximately 30 minutes, then the catheter is opened up and the fluid is drained out. Since the peritoneal dialysis replaces your kidney function, routine blood work must be drawn to make sure the dialysis is working effectively.

As always, I'll give you some risk vs. reward to consider. The benefit of dialysis is life. One benefit of peritoneal as opposed to hemodialysis is that you may be able to do the peritoneal dialysis by yourself at home. We already discussed the reasons why, without kidney function, you will die. The alternative is dialysis and if you can tolerate the lifestyle changes you can live a long life. As we have covered with each topic, there are also risks involved. Peritoneal dialysis has a great risk of infection. The catheter goes right through your skin and it is an easy target for bacteria. If the bacteria causes a bad enough infection, the catheter will be removed and you may have to have the second type of dialysis, hemodialysis. Other side effects may include hernia or fluid leaking into the scrotum on males. Even less likely, but a risk nonetheless, is that you may be allergic to the dialysis fluid that gets poured into your body.

Hemodialysis is the more invasive of the two dialysis procedures. This involves removing your blood, pumping it through an artificial kidney and then returning it to your body. That is the very basic idea of it, but let me clarify that not ALL your blood is taken out at the same time. They estimate that only about a cup of blood is out of your body at one time. Hemodialysis usually takes two to five hours and will be regularly scheduled as much as every day or as little as once a week, depending on the severity of your condition. This is typically done in your doctor's office or at a dialysis clinic where you will have dialysis with a few other dialysis patients. Many of the people on dialysis say it helps a lot to meet and talk with other people going through the same things they are. It can become a kind of support group.

In most cases, a dialysis access 'graft' is permanently placed in your arm or leg, allowing for easy connection to the dialysis machine. The dialysis graft is a man made tube that is sewn between an artery and a vein. Your blood then flows from the artery to the vein. It is this graft that they access to take out your blood for dialysis. This is easier on you, the patient, because there is less chance of damage to your blood vessels when the blood is taken out.

Of course there is always the risk reward to consider for hemodialysis. Once again, the obvious benefit to having hemodialysis is that it can help to keep you alive.

However, there are many risk factors. As we have discussed numerous times before, infection is the most common risk. Every time they access your dialysis graft there is the chance of getting a bacterial infection. Another risk is a drop in your blood pressure. This is not as severe of a risk. However, if you have heart problems too, a drop in blood pressure could make dialysis difficult on your heart. When you have dialysis you are given a blood

thinner, heparin for example. You will want to avoid
shaving or any activity that involves the risk of
being cut or bleeding for a few hours after dialysis.
Because of the blood thinner, it will be very hard to
stop you from bleeding should you cut yourself.
You can see that there are many risks, but again, it
may be worth it if dialysis can save your life.

In my experience, people that have peritoneal
dialysis have a shorter recovery period, as opposed
to patients that have had hemodialysis who are
pretty wiped out for a few hours afterward. The
good thing about hemodialysis is that you go once
in a day and it is over. Peritoneal may have to be
performed four to five times a day because it is less
effective.

The other treatment of kidney failure is the
most obvious -- kidney transplant. It is not like
kidneys are readily available though and you may
need some type of dialysis to sustain you until a
donor kidney can be found. If a family member or
loved one has the same blood type, they can decide
to donate a kidney to you. There is less of a wait in
that case. In the case that you are waiting for a
donor who has recently died, you may wait months
or years for your new kidney depending on your
blood type.

There are very strict guidelines for kidney
transplant, and not everyone will qualify for a
transplant. Your doctor will go over specific health
guidelines for you and your donor. If you do qualify,
the surgery will be performed as soon as possible. If
you are waiting for a donor kidney from someone
who has died, you will be on standby. On standby

you may get a call that they've got a kidney for you. In which case, you will have been given instructions on what to do when the call comes in. It becomes a race against time to get the new kidney into you in the shortest amount of time possible, so you must be ready to go!

Once at the hospital, a kidney transplant can take three to six hours. There are just a couple of notes about kidney transplant that I'd like to share with you. First, your old kidneys will not be removed. Second, the new kidney will be tested for disease before it is transplanted. Lastly, your new kidney might work immediately or it might not start working for a week or two. As with any transplant, you will be placed on medication that suppresses your immune system. This is so your body doesn't attack the new kidney, because your body will view it only as a foreign body that doesn't belong there. But you will have to take the immune suppression medications for the rest of your life.

So here we are once again at our risk vs. reward review. As we have stated before, your life is at stake and that is the reward for risking a kidney transplant. There are of course, the risks. First, there is the surgery. Any time you have a major surgery there is the risk of infection, internal bleeding, pneumonia, or having a reaction to the anesthesia. Then there is the risk that your body might reject the new kidney. In which case the new kidney may no longer work, it will be removed and you will need dialysis. (You may also get on the list for a second kidney transplant.) Lastly, there are the effects of taking drugs that hold back your immune system. That means you will be more likely to have colds, infections, and various pneumonia, all of which will be more severe than what you are used to because your body can't fight them as well as it used to.

The kidneys are complicated and life-sustaining organs. You can see why they need some attention in this book. You can also see why I would direct you to a Nephrologist for more in depth questions regarding kidney failure. On the bright side, there aren't many treatment options to learn because there is no treatment. There is only replacement of kidney function. How you go about filtering your blood should you have kidney failure should be included in your Living Will. You and your spouse may want to discuss whether or not you would want to donate a kidney to the other. You may even go so far as to find out what blood types you are because you may not be compatible.

I'd like to add one quick side note before we finish Mr. Wayne's story. The easiest and cheapest way to figure out your blood type is to go donate blood. There is ALWAYS a shortage of blood and you may save someone's life. Giving blood only takes a few minutes and you will probably only feel a little weak for a couple of hours, but the rewards are endless! Give blood today.

Mr. Wayne's situation is a pretty simple case as far as kidney failure goes. His kidneys were starting to shut down and the symptom that was most easily noticed was his breathing. As we learned in this chapter, the kidneys have an affect on many different bodily functions, one of which is regulating blood pH. That is, how acidic the blood is. Because of that, his breathing was affected. As we learned, we breathe out carbon dioxide. Carbon Dioxide is an acid when it is in your blood. The kidneys regulate blood pH by making a base to counteract the acidic carbon dioxide.

When Mr. Wayne's kidney's stopped making the base, the pH in his blood became more acidic. His body was then trying to normalize the pH of the blood by removing as much carbon dioxide as possible, by hyperventilating. Mr. Wayne came in because he was breathing too fast in order to remove carbon dioxide, to normalize his blood pH, because his kidneys were failing.

Mr. Wayne received a few dialysis treatments while at the hospital. His breathing returned to normal and he was sent back to his long-term care facility. He will have dialysis every other day for the rest of his life. Mr. Wayne was not a candidate for a kidney transplant because he was very close to life expectancy for the mentally retarded and he was already on life sustaining treatment (the ventilator).

Your "Kidney Failure" Checklist:

Now that we've covered these medical treatments
that help to do the work of the kidneys, it is time to
make your choice. Which of the following will you
want and which do you prefer not to have?

>Peritoneal Dialysis
        (Fluid poured into your abdomen then taken
        out)

>Hemodialysis
        (Blood is removed, filtered and pumped back
        in.)

>Transplant
        (A new kidney is placed in your body.)

Food

It is estimated that the average American eats
1,500 pounds of food each year.

Mr. Silver was a 74-year-old retired gentleman. He was very active around his house, particularly in his garden. You see, Mr. Silver had immigrated to America as a teenager and loved to grow flowers, fruits and vegetables from his native Portugal. It goes without saying that he loved his wife's cooking, especially when she used his home-grown ingredients. Mr. Silver had gone to see his doctor because he was coughing, "only when he ate." The doctor ordered some tests with the local Speech Pathologist. The speech people are also experts on swallowing, so they are the ones to see for speech and or swallowing problems. Before the day of Mr. Silver's appointment to see his speech pathologist, he was admitted to my ward because he was having difficulty breathing. He was diagnosed with pneumonia. It seems that Mr. Silva was coughing while he ate because some of the food was getting into his lungs.

Food is the provider of energy for our bodies. Like breathing, the heart and kidney function, we all know that we need to eat to live. The next question then becomes why someone wouldn't be able to eat. There are many reasons why, but typically the reasons can all be broken down into two categories. Either someone is physically unable to eat, or when they do eat the food goes down the wrong pipe into the lungs. An example of why someone physically can't eat is the treatment we give them when they can't breathe. The Endotracheal tube is taped into their mouth so there is no way they can chew and swallow food. The example of someone who swallows down the wrong pipe gets a little more complicated and will require some explanation.

Our anatomy for swallowing has a built-in design flaw. Some have called it nature's way of limiting our lifespan. Our anatomy is designed so that the air we breathe and the food we eat all start in the same tube, an area known as the pharynx (pronounced fair-inks) behind the nose and mouth. (You may remember this from our discussion about the AMBU bag.) The pharynx can be further divided into two sections. The upper pharynx where air comes in through your nose is called the nasopharynx and the lower portion where the food would enter is called the oropharynx. From there, the pharynx separates into two tubes, one to the lungs and one to the stomach. This is the design flaw I mentioned. When you choke, food has gone toward the lungs instead of stomach. To help with this problem, there is a 'valve' where the pharynx splits in two called the epiglottis. The job of this valve is to ensure that air and or food go into the correct tube.

Typically, the epiglottis covers the tube to the stomach because we are always breathing. This ensures that the air we breathe in goes to the lungs. When we swallow food, the epiglottis covers our airway and the food is pushed down toward the stomach. But what if someone's epiglottis stops working or just doesn't work as well as it used to? It is very common for the elderly to have problems swallowing and the older you get the more likely the epiglottis is to fail. Now you have a better understanding of the second reason why someone wouldn't be able to eat, the food going down the wrong pipe. The medical term for food going down the wrong pipe is called aspiration. You may also hear it called aspirating, aspirated or aspirate. The next logical question is:

What can be done about it?

For the normal, healthy person who has developed a problem swallowing there are some helpful therapies. There is even an entire medical field devoted to it, the Speech and Language Pathologist. Problems swallowing are generally caused by the consistency of what you are eating. For instance, the consistency of water is thin, whereas the consistency of honey is thick. You are more likely to aspirate water than honey. The thicker the consistency, the more likely the epiglottis will be able to cover your airway. The Speech and Language Pathologists also have some swallowing techniques that help the anatomy to do its job properly. These include sitting upright, swallowing twice or tucking your chin to your chest when you swallow. There is a progression that occurs as the swallowing gets worse.

If all of the above therapies do not help, and you still get food in your lungs when you eat, then we must seek an alternate solution. That solution is in the form of a feeding tube. When it is decided that you need a feeding tube, they first place a temporary tube to see if you will tolerate it. The temporary tube is known as a Naso-Gastric or NG Tube. The NG tube is placed through your nose, through the pharynx where you are asked to swallow the tube. The tube is then passed down your esophagus into the stomach. Lastly, the feeding tube is then taped to your nose so it doesn't come out. A feeding tube like this is also used when you have the breathing tube in your lungs because you are on a ventilator and cannot physically swallow. That allows you to get nutrition while on the breathing machine and when you no longer need the ventilator the temporary feeding tube can also be taken out. If the NG tube must be a long-term solution, surgery is needed.

Before that, we must touch on the risk and reward for the NG Tube. Obviously, the reward is that you are receiving much needed nutrition. Some risks include trauma to the back of the throat or esophagus, nose bleeds, and of course, infection. All are pretty minor, but something to consider.

The next step in the process is where another major medical decision is made. The decision to have a permanent feeding tube placed usually becomes the moment of truth for our patients. This is very similar to the endotracheal tube being replaced with a trach tube, in that it is another major decision for you or your loved ones. It is at this point that some decide not to have the procedure done. Most people are comfortable with the idea of a temporary feeding tube. It becomes a big decision for most people to go permanent. A controversy in Florida may help to illustrate why this is such a big decision.

The most popular example in recent history about the use of a feeding tube as life support is the Terry Schiavo case.[1] Where do we even begin with this one? Everyone has already chosen a side on the Schiavo case. The fact is that she could not eat and she had a permanent feeding tube keeping her alive. The problem was that she never made it clear IN WRITING whether or not she would want to be kept alive that way. She told her husband that she didn't, or at least that was his story. You already know the controversy it caused. Her husband didn't want her to go on living with a feeding tube and her parents wanted her to be fed. Obviously, without being fed she would die from lack of nutrition. The question no one could answer was if she was really "alive" anyway. She blinked and seemed to smile, but could not write or talk or communicate. For all they knew, she might have understood fully what

---

[1] Quill, Timoth E. M.D. "Terry Schiavo -- A Tragecy Compounded." New England Journal of Medicine. www.nejm.org. April 21, 2005.

was going on. For all they knew, she may have had no thought at all. This is a good case to use for an example because just about everyone is familiar with it. Please talk to your loved ones and explain to them that you don't want to be the next Schiavo case. Make it clear to everyone that you want to be fed or you don't want to live with a permanent feeding tube.

The permanent feeding tube is called a PEG Tube. This is short for (and you're not expected to be able to say this) Percutaneous Endoscopic Gastrostomy. The procedure itself is a minor surgery and I've literally watched it performed right in patient's rooms. Essentially, the surgeon puts a scope in your mouth down to the stomach. The scope has a light on the end of it so the surgeon can see where it is in the body. When it is in the right place, an 'x' is marked on the skin over the stomach where the light is. The scope is pulled back and an incision is made through the skin and into the stomach. The feed tube is then secured into the stomach through the hole, it is stitched up and feeding can begin. So rather than a feeding tube through your nose and into your stomach you have a tube coming directly out of your stomach. For someone who can no longer eat, this is more beneficial.

Let's say you had cancer and your epiglottis was removed so you can no longer eat. If you have a PEG tube, you can be home and live a normal life. You'd be able to go out in public and no one would have any clue that you have a PEG. When mealtime comes, you simply pour the food into your tube.

Let's not get carried away here, you aren't eating pork chops and gravy.

Tube feed comes in cans and since you never taste it, it is not made to taste good. The tube feed comes in different formulas depending on your nutritional needs. Some have high fiber, some have high protein, etc. Tube feeding can be done one of two ways. Normally in the hospital setting an amount is given over time, so three or four cans may be given continuously over eight to 10 hours. It may also be given all at once which is known as a bolus feeding. This is more feasible for someone living at home with a PEG tube.

The risk/reward is pretty easy for tube feeding. The reward is that you are fed and kept alive. The risks are pretty minimal. Besides the usual infections, risks include not tolerating the food and routine blood tests to make sure you get the proper nutrition.

There is also a third method of receiving nutrition. This is for people with stomach or intestinal problems that cannot digest food or simply cannot tolerate tube feedings. In this case, nutrition is given directly into the blood stream. Total Parenteral Nutrition (TPN for short) is a precise mixture of nutrients given through an IV site directly into your blood. Your doctor will prescribe a specific list of nutrients that you will need to receive and how much of each you should get. A pharmacist then puts the mixture together shortly before it is given to you. In most cases a long-term IV must be placed, one that can stay in for six weeks or more without having to be changed.

When the IV bag containing the mixture is ready, it will be attached to your long term IV site. It usually takes 10-12 hours for the entire mixture to enter your blood. Most often TPN will be given at night while you are sleeping so that you don't have to be attached to an IV all day long.

There are also cases where TPN can be administered by you or your loved one if you need to have it at home. In this case you will also do the TPN overnight. You will be taught how to attach it to your IV and what side effects to watch out for. That leads us nicely in to our risk vs. reward for TPN.

I hope that you are not tired of reading the reward as staying alive, because that is the reward for using TPN. There are not typically any side effects, except those that go along with having an IntraVenous line. That is, infection, skin irritation and having to change the IV site. Again, you will have blood drawn on a regular basis to ensure that you are getting proper nutrition.

Mr. Silver's specific diagnosis was aspiration pneumonia, which is the fancy term for food going down the wrong pipe and into the lungs. Work with the speech pathologist showed that he was not swallowing properly. No matter what consistency they tried, Mr. Silver aspirated. Next they brought him to have an x-ray of him swallowing. The x-ray revealed that the anatomy of Mr. Silver's throat was not normal. An ear, nose and throat doctor, "E.N.T." was brought in to see him. An E.N.T. is a surgeon, and most commonly they like to look inside people to see exactly what's going on. The

E.N.T. put a scope down Mr. Silver's throat and visualized several masses of flesh. That is, flesh that has grown abnormally or which should not be there in the first place. The E.N.T. took a sample of a couple of these masses for testing that revealed cancer. An MRI showed many more masses up and down Mr. Silver's throat, too many to operate on successfully. For the foreseeable future, he would not be able to eat. Mr. Silver had an NG tube inserted until treatment for his cancer could be decided upon and started.

Mr. Silver began having his cancer treatments and they weren't helping very much. He became confused and agitated. In addition, he kept pulling the NG feeding tube out of his nose. His breathing got worse, and upon further inspection, the ENT surgeon saw that the masses were starting to block his airway. Mr. Silver's family decided to have the tracheostomy procedure performed on him in order to keep his airway open while he continued cancer treatment. During several weeks of treatment in which time he pulled out his NG tube upwards of 20 times, it was decided that Mr. Silver would get a PEG tube for his feeding. The NG tube was taken out for the last time and a surgeon inserted the PEG tube into Mr. Silver's stomach. His feedings were done at night while he was sleeping and the PEG tube was kept tucked into an abdominal binder during the day, so he wouldn't be tempted to pull it out. When Mr. Silver finally left the hospital, he couldn't go home because his elderly wife was unable to handle all the facets of his care. He still had a trach tube and a PEG tube, which meant he needed to be suctioned constantly and fed through his PEG tube. Mr. Silver was transferred to a long-term care facility where he passed away after a few weeks.

Your "Food" Checklist:

You've read about the three methods of being fed or obtaining nutrition, once again it is time to make your decision. Which of the following will you want and which do you prefer to not have?

>Nasogastric Tube
        (the tube up your nose and into the stomach)

>Percutaneous Endoscopic Gastrostomy
        (tube directly in stomach)

>Total Parenteral Nutrition
        (IV Feedings)

To Be or Not To Be

Quality of Life

"You are not truly prepared to live until you are prepared to die."
                                        - Dr. Charles Stanley

This chapter will focus on some things that may or may not be put in writing in your Living Will. The life-saving medical procedures you've learned about so far are pretty clear. The decisions about them are probably just yes and no. Therefore, they are the procedures your doctor will ask you about at your bedside and the ones your estate planning attorney will ask you about in order to prepare your Living Will. This chapter, which is titled "Quality of Life," is really focused on some of the other things you may want to consider when making your medical decisions.

Death is one of the hardest things to talk about, yet also one of the most important topics you should discuss with your spouse. Both should write their individual wishes in a Living Will. Failure to talk about these and other considerations may result in a death that you never wanted, or you may put a lot of stress on a loved one to make these tough decisions for you.

In this chapter, I will include some common situations that occur both when you decide to use

life support, and when you decide not to be saved.
These other issues should be considered when you
make your decision whether or not to have life-
saving procedures.

In order to best divide the miscellaneous
topics, I feel it is best to break them down into two
categories. The first category will be for those who
feel like they would like to be kept alive by the life-
sustaining medical treatments. The second category
is for those people who feel they do not want to be
kept alive by superficial means. In either case,
there are consequences that accompany those
decisions.

If you have made up your mind that you
would like to be kept alive, the following topics will
be of particular concern. Even if you decide that
you do not want life-saving medical procedures, you
may encounter some of these issues. I will speak in
generalities, because there are so many different
reasons which may require life-saving medical
procedures, I cannot cover everything. It would take
volumes of medical books and most of it would be
disease states or conditions that I could not even
pronounce, never mind speak of with any
knowledge.

First, consider where you will live. This can
get complicated because depending on what
medical treatment is keeping you alive, if any, you
may be able to go home. In the Kidneys chapter we
learned that you may live at home and simply
report to your local dialysis center for treatments
every other day. But if your kidney failure is severe,
you will have other complications that may require

being in the hospital or some other skilled nursing facility. Also, depending upon your medical condition and residence, your insurance company may dictate a course of action.

For example, Mrs. Shaw was on a ventilator at the hospital. Her kids were grown and had families of their own and jobs to worry about. Mrs. Shaw could not care for herself at home and her family was also unable to care for her. Her insurance would only cover one hour of daily nurse visits to her home. Yet there was no way that Mrs. Shaw could be home alone 23 hours a day. She could not prepare meals, wash herself or use the commode on her own. She needed someone's help with each. The next logical step then, is to go to some sort of nursing home where there is staffing 24 hours a day to help with such daily activities.

A nursing home may also be called a skilled nursing facility. Due to the way they get paid by insurance companies, most "nursing homes" refer to themselves as some type of "rehabilitation center" these days. In the end though, that is what it is. A nursing home is a business like any other -- and each is very selective about who is admitted.

The nursing homes, rehabilitation centers, long-term care centers and hospitals alike are under tremendous financial strain. Nurses make these places work. Without nurses there would be no medical facilities. The problem is, there is a severe nursing shortage. In order to hire and retain nurses, medical facilities have to pay top dollar. They are also under federal guidelines as to how

many nurses they need to have on staff for each
shift.

In addition, insurance companies only pay
what they feel a medical treatment is worth. For
instance, the hospital performs a chest x-ray on
you for possible pneumonia. The hospital has to
pay for the x-ray room, the x-ray machine,
maintenance of the machine, supplies for the
machine, a radiology technician to perform the x-
ray and a doctor (Radiologist) to read the x-ray. For
all of that, let's just say the hospital bills your
insurance company $200. (I do not know the actual
charge.)

Well, your insurance company deems that a
chest x-ray for someone with pneumonia is only
worth $125. The hospital loses $75 and tries to bill
it to the patient. But if the patient doesn't pay, it's
probably not worth the legal fees to try to get the
$75 back. This is only one example, but you can
see how fragile the finances of medical facilities can
be.

So when it comes to admitting a patient to a
nursing home, the patient whose insurance
company pays the most will be the one accepted. It
is sad, but so very true.

There was no facility willing to accept Mrs.
Shaw. The cost of care for a person on a ventilator
is way too high for a medical facility. If they
accepted her, they would lose thousands of dollars
every month. So Mrs. Shaw had to stay in the
hospital, in her room for two years before she
passed away. She stayed in the same room, same

four walls, same view, never leaving the room, and certainly never going outside.

Some insurance companies today sell long-term care insurance to help pay for future medical housing, such as a nursing home. Whether or not you're thinking that you'd like to be kept alive, make sure that you at least explore the option of long-term care insurance.

Another way to pay for long-term care is with your home. If you own a home, it can be sold and the proceeds are then used to pay the medical facility where you would live. If you are in a facility and your insurance coverage runs out, the facility may try to force you to sell your home. But what if that is where your spouse lives? Your spouse may not be forced to sell, but a lien may be put on the home to pay the medical bills once the house is eventually sold.

So just thinking about where you are going to live can get very complicated. Again, depending on what medical treatments you require to keep you alive, you can live in your home, in a long-term facility, a nursing home or even in the hospital. Talk with your loved ones, and perhaps your financial planner and estate attorney about future housing options.

Another topic that should be discussed is mobility. Are you able to walk? Do you need a mechanical or electric wheelchair, perhaps both? Can you move at all? Again, for something as simple as a feeding tube, in an uncomplicated situation, you may not only be home but also healthy enough to have a job. Under other health circumstances, you may become bedridden.

Mrs. Shaw walked into the emergency room. Even on the ventilator, she could walk short distances. She would get up and sit in a chair for meals, and was able to walk to a commode. But as her condition deteriorated, she no could longer get out of bed. She spent the last six months of her life in her hospital bed.

Your doctor should be able to give you and or your loved ones some idea of how mobile you could be given your specific health issues. While the idea of having to use a wheelchair is not anyone's first choice, it beats having to stay in bed all day. If you will be bedridden, possibly unconscious or unable to use a wheelchair on your own, you may be placed in a chair during the day, or you may even be able to go outside if you are medically stable enough. Great advancements have been made in the rehabilitation fields in last couple of decades. As I mentioned, many nursing homes now offer some level of rehab. You may improve your mobility with some rehab work to where you could go home and care for yourself.

The next topic deals with patients who have very limited or no mobility. There is no shame or humility for patients in medical facilities. If you cannot move from your bed, or you have limited ability to move, you will be washed daily by a member of the medical staff. Males will be washed by male or female staff and females will be washed by male or female staff. And then there is the issue of going to the bathroom. Regardless of medical condition, people still move their bowels every day and people still urinate every day. There are many different ways to use the facilities when you have to go. If you are bedridden and not conscious enough to call for help, you'll lie there in bed and move your bowels in bed and wait until the staff notice it and clean you. You may also be in an adult diaper. If you are bedridden but you can ring the call light for help, the staff will place a bedpan under you. With a little ability to move, you may sit on a commode at your bedside. With better mobility you may actually get to walk to the bathroom. It's not something that we think so much about during the course of our normal adult life, but most of us like our privacy when we use the bathroom or take a shower. This privacy may be taken away if you cannot move well enough while having life sustaining medical treatment.

Another issue to think about involves how well you can move yourself. More specifically, consider those who are bedridden, and the issue is bed sores.

I'd like you to participate in a little experiment to help me illustrate what I'm writing about. I want you to go lie down in bed for a few minutes. Take your shoes off and lie flat on your back. You can use a pillow if you need it. Place your arms by your sides and keep your legs uncrossed. Now see how long you can lie there without moving. The most I've done is about 25 minutes before I had to move. You'll feel pressure points where the weight of your body is supported by the mattress. The first place you feel the pressure is in your

heels. Then you feel your bottom start to go numb.
Go ahead and try it. If you lasted 25 minutes, I'm
impressed.

The point is, bedridden means in bed all day
every day. The medical staff will usually turn you
from one side to the other about every two hours.
That's two HOURS, not 25 minutes. When you start
to feel discomfort in your heels and bottom, it is
because there is less circulation to those areas.
That is when bed sores start to form. The weight of
your body pressing into the mattress squishes your
little blood vessels in those areas. Lack of
circulation leads to lack of oxygen to the skin cells
in your heel and bottom. The lack of oxygen slowly
kills the skin cells. It starts with a red area where
the skin has been in contact with the bed. As time
goes on, the dead skin starts to break down,
exposing the tissue underneath the skin. The tissue
dies and turns black. The area can get larger and
larger. I have seen with my own eyes, bed sores big
enough to put my fist in. Needless to say an open
wound that you're lying on is very painful. I'm not
trying to say that bed sores happen to everyone
who can't get out of bed. New air mattress beds and
special creams as well as better staff awareness
have all reduced the number of cases of bed sores.
The fact remains though, that bed sores do occur
and you should be aware of them.

Early on in Mrs. Shaw's hospital stay, she
was out of bed a lot. As she got worse, she was in
bed more and more. As red areas began to form bed
sores, we used a special air mattress on her bed.
The staff also became more aware of turning her

from side to side more regularly. Fortunately, her skin never broke out into bed sores, but she did have pretty large red areas that had to be very uncomfortable. Of course, she lost her ability to speak, so I'm not really sure if her red areas were painful or not.

## Ability to Communicate

This leads us to the next topic: you may or may not be able to communicate. There are different levels of communication. If you are being kept alive with dialysis for instance, you'll probably be able to talk. At other times you are being kept alive, you may not be conscious. And still other times, you may be fully aware of your surroundings but cannot talk. You may be able to write your needs on paper. If you cannot talk or write, you can point to letters or pictures of what you need.

For some people, the idea of being fully conscious without being able to talk or communicate is a nightmare. For others, the security of still being alive makes not being able to communicate worth it. If you remember the Terry Schiavo case, she could not communicate at all. She couldn't talk, write or point to things. She was being kept alive by a feeding tube. Her husband thought that she had had enough and wanted to remove the tube and let her die. Her parents, on the other hand, felt like she knew when they were there and that she might be fully conscious but not able to communicate. This is the main reason why you should put your wishes in writing; you probably don't want to put your spouse and or parents in a similar situation. Terry Schiavo's feeding was stopped and an autopsy later revealed that she was not aware of what was going on.

Eating on Your Own

We've already covered the options for you about the feeding tube, but you should also consider whether or not you will be able to eat. It doesn't sound like a big deal, but to some of you it is a very big deal. I have met patients who decided that they never want a feeding tube, and never want a PEG. They choose to eat, even though some of the food they swallow ends up in their lungs, which could eventually kill them. In their minds, they would rather die than be told they can not eat their favorite foods.

We've gone over quite a few other topics for your consideration. The purpose of pointing them out is not to try to talk you out of being kept alive. The purpose was to stay within the guidelines of this book, and give you as much information as possible, good or bad, so that you can make a better informed decision. If you have weighed all the facts and you personally feel that you'd rather not be kept alive by artificial means, put it in writing. Every person that gets admitted to the hospital is asked if they would like to be kept alive. When the answer is no, the person is a DNR -- Do Not Resuscitate. The "DNR" order from your doctor is placed in writing in your chart and the staff is made aware of it.

A DNR order does not mean you will not be given medical treatment. For instance, if you take pills to control your blood pressure, they will still be given. If you are diabetic, your blood sugar will still be monitored and treated accordingly. A DNR simply means that if your heart stops and or you stop breathing on your own, you will not be revived. Instead of breathing for you and possibly shocking your heart as we have previously discussed, the medical personnel will let you die.

Preparing for the Inevitable: The Stages of Death and Dying

Eventually we all die. I didn't need to tell you that. No matter what heroic methods are used, the human body is still designed to, and will, die. The next section will be about some options you may have in death. The doctor comes to you (or your loved ones on your behalf) to tell you that it's your time. The doctor may also estimate how long you have to live. The common story is someone is diagnosed with cancer and given six months to live, or maybe one year. When the doctor can see the end in sight and imparts that information to you, he or she tells you so that you can prepare to die according to your wishes.

But what is your condition when the word comes? You may not have much of a choice except to die in the hospital bed with machines attached. It may be that the machines will be stopped so you can die -- "pulling the plug" as it is sometimes called. Maybe it's a Terry Schiavo situation where your feeding tube will be removed. The point is that you may not have any choice about where or how you die. If you are given a choice, you may want to give the following topics some consideration.

In this section the option becomes where will you die. A lot of people want to be home. There's not only something about being home when you're healthy, but also something about being home when you're terminally ill. Some people are too sick and choose to stay in the hospital to have symptoms treated. If you are living in a nursing home, you may pass away there. You should check the nursing home's policy on dying residents before choosing a nursing home. Many times nursing home patients are sent to the emergency room because they are dying.

This is a typical scenario from my viewpoint. An 88-year-old woman has lost consciousness, so the nursing home has her rushed to the hospital in an ambulance. The family is contacted and they say they do not want life support for her. She gets admitted to my unit where we give her some oxygen and her normal meds, and she is allowed to pass away. Sometimes she doesn't die and goes back to the nursing home as an unconscious resident.

Another consideration at the end of your life is what sort of treatments you want. This can also get tricky. You may have options about oxygen, pain medications and hydration. More than likely, these options will still exist whether you choose to die at home or in a medical setting. Let's take a closer look at each.

One of the first symptoms that death is near is a change from the regular breathing pattern. The change in breathing leads to less oxygen being breathed into your lungs. Normally, when oxygen levels fall, supplemental oxygen is given. Oxygen can be given quite comfortably through a cannula or a mask. An oxygen cannula is a small clear, pliable tube that wraps behind the ears and has two prongs that go into each nostril. A flow of oxygen runs through the tubing into your nose and you breathe in extra oxygen. Most people are content with supplemental oxygen. Some feel that it just prolongs the inevitable and choose not to have it. There is no right or wrong here, but oxygen will generally be given unless you specify you do not want it.

Another consideration is whether or not you'd like pain medication. This may vary greatly depending on the reason you are dying. In the case of the 88-year-old from the nursing home, because she's older, her body is naturally shutting down and she's probably not experiencing much pain. There may be other situations, such as some types of cancer that are very painful. You may need to play it by ear and have pain meds only with pain. One problem is that at some point you go unconscious, and then no one knows how much pain you are in, or if you are even experiencing pain at all.

Another problem is that the pain medications tend to slow down life functions. For example, morphine slows down your breathing. The struggle that most pharmacists have is that, while pain meds take away the pain, they may also be killing you. It's a very delicate balance, and it is hard to know where to draw the line between taking away pain and actually speeding up the dying process.

Another end of life topic, one that has been greatly debated, is hydration. That is, whether or not you get water. "Get water" is a tricky issue and it goes beyond just wetting your lips if you are thirsty. You can wet your lips if you're thirsty or your mouth is dry. If the situation arises that you are unable to drink for any reason, you must decide whether or not you want fluids through an intravenous (IV) line. The great debate about hydration is being argued on two fronts.

Those that are in favor of hydration argue that it is cruel to die from dehydration (lack of water). They make a case that the fluids help with mental status. That is patients that receive fluids tend to be less agitated, have reduced confusion and less restlessness. Those in favor of hydration also make the point that fluids help prevent the kidneys from shutting down.

Those that are against hydration argue that dehydration is not painful and may be more humane than giving IV fluids. In addition to breathing changes, when your body is shutting down, the heart does not beat as efficiently. They argue that fluids can overload your body causing further medical complications. Extra fluid can stress the failing heart. Extra fluid can also end up in the lungs, making it harder to breathe. As these parts of the body shut down, they argue, you want to let them shut down, not work them harder.

Excess fluid may also cause swelling in the arms and legs as well as around tumors. This swelling can be very painful.

Hydration decisions can be made on a case by case basis. Looking at both sides, they each have valid points. Once again, depending on your situation, what is causing your death may dictate whether or not you should receive fluids. They are sometimes optional, though, so you should give it some thought.

Finally, you should consider what else you might want when it is YOU who is dying. You may not be given any choices about death, but you may have some time to plan and control your surroundings. Some people want their family around, while others would rather be alone. Who do you want to visit while you are dying and who do you not want around you? Some people choose to have particular types of music or certain favorite artists' music playing in the background. Some people like the lights on and others would rather have it be dark. It is your choice and if you are fortunate enough to have a choice, you should make the most of it. Ask for whatever you think you need to make your passing easiest for you. All of these options and issues can be spelled out for your loved ones and your doctor in your Living Will.

In Summary

I cannot stress to you enough the main reason why I wrote this book.

That reason can be summed up in one word – *anguish.*

For nearly 20 years I have worked on the front lines of death and dying. I have saved countless lives and I have pulled the plug on numerous others. I have had my hand in someone's chest performing chest compressions by literally squeezing his heart in my hands. In experiencing family members over the years, in most cases they can come to terms with the fact that their spouse or parent is dying. But what they never get over, what they anguish over is making decisions for their loved one. On too many occasions to count, a teary eyed son or daughter turns to me and expresses how they hope they are doing the right thing. They don't know what their loved one would have wanted and now the decision is on them. That anguish becomes harder to deal with than the actual death.

It is for them that I toiled over this book and took on the expense of self-publishing it. There is no reason why anyone should ever have to go through the pain and suffering of deciding whether or not to keep a parent or spouse alive. Or whether or not to have critical and sometimes painful procedures performed on them.

The one thing I have learned in my experiences is that you MUST speak with your spouse and your children or next of kin about the issues I have presented in this book. You should put those wishes in writing, but at the absolute, very least talk about it with them. I do not want to see another person go through that anguish. Please pass the word.

## Appendix A:  A Summary of Checklists from Each Chapter

Your "Breathing" Checklist:

>AMBU (the bag that simulates mouth to mouth)
>BiPAP (the machine that breathes for you without a tube)
>Intubation (the tube in your mouth and vocal chords)
>Ventilator (breathing machine with intubation tube)
>Tracheostomy (hole in neck with shorter breathing tube)


Your "Heart" Checklist:

>Compressions (a person pushing down on your chest)
>Defibrillation (shocking your heart with electricity)
>Cardiac Meds (help change the way the heart pumps)

Your "Kidney Failure" Checklist:

>Peritoneal Dialysis (Fluid poured into your abdomen)
>Hemodialysis (Blood is removed, filtered and put back in.)
>Transplant (A new kidney is placed in your body.)

Your "Food" Checklist:

>Nasogastric Tube (the tube in nose and into the stomach)
>Percutaneous Endoscopic Gastrostomy (tube in stomach)
>Total Parenteral Nutrition (IV Feedings)